Movement Skills

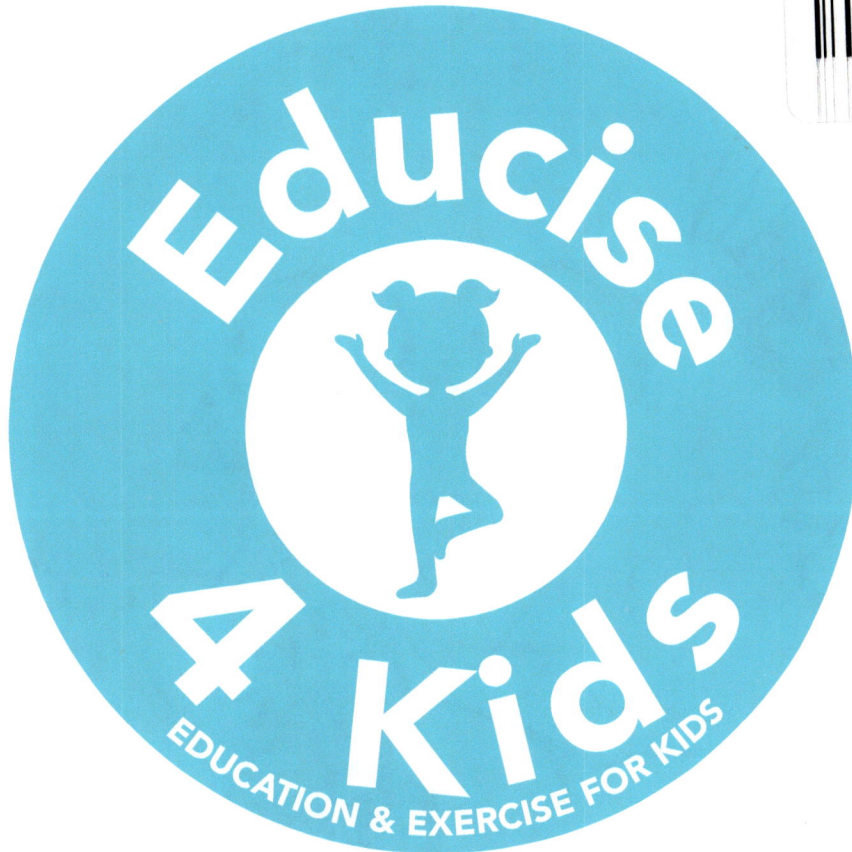

Educise
4 Kids
EDUCATION & EXERCISE FOR KIDS

Created By
Priscilla Fauvette

Illustrated By
Bernard Fauvette

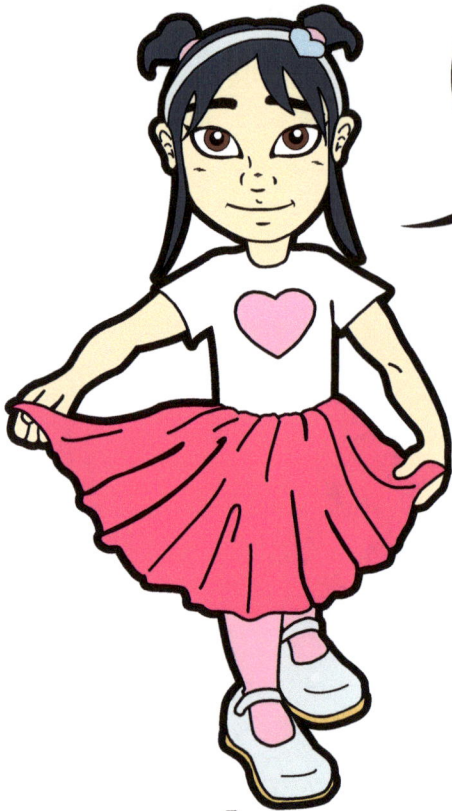

MAKE TIME FOR REST & RELAXATION

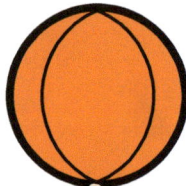

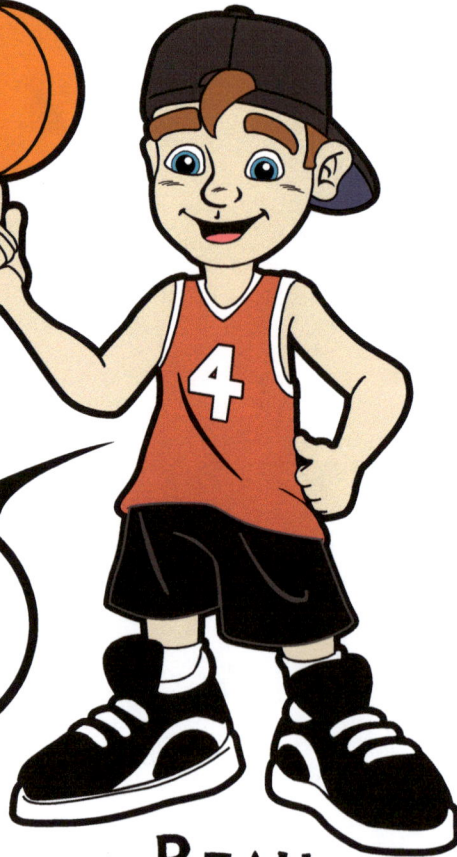

LIN

DRINK PLENTY OF WATER

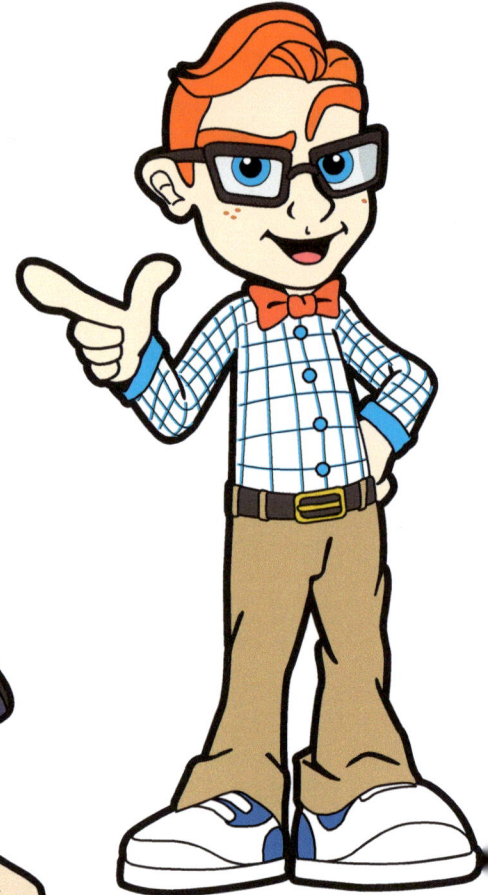

BEAU

CADEN

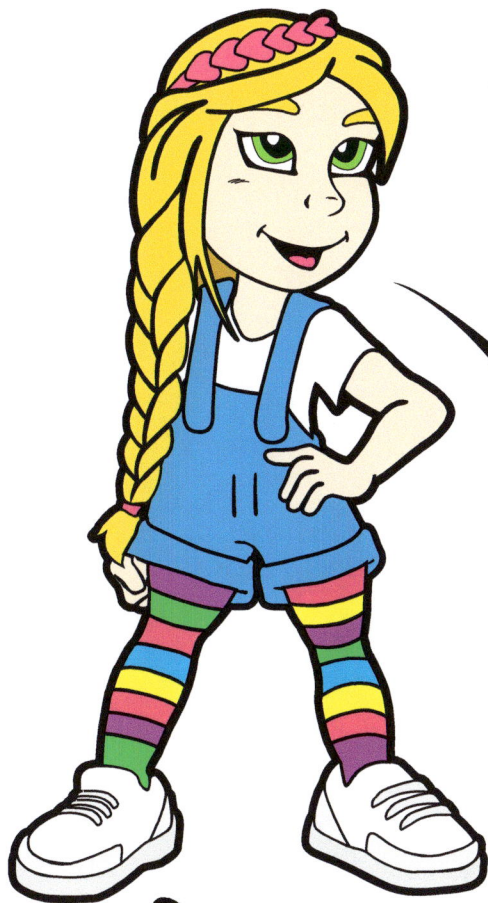

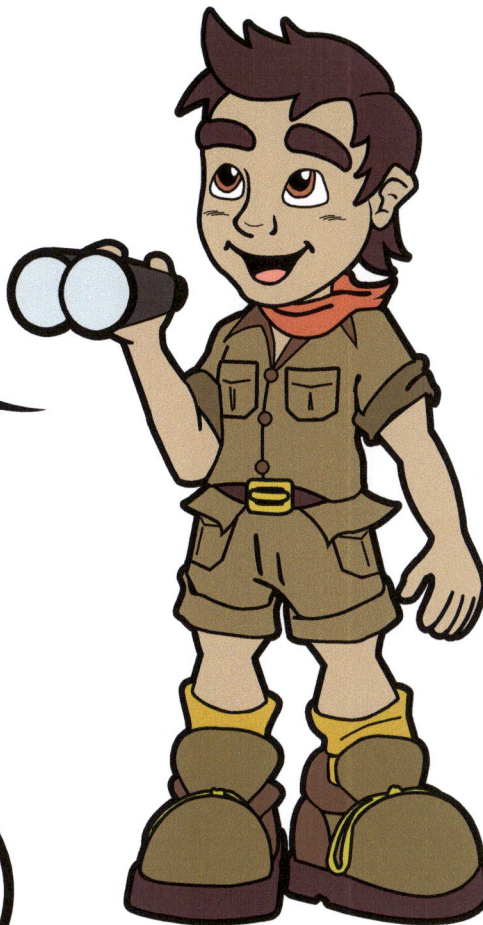

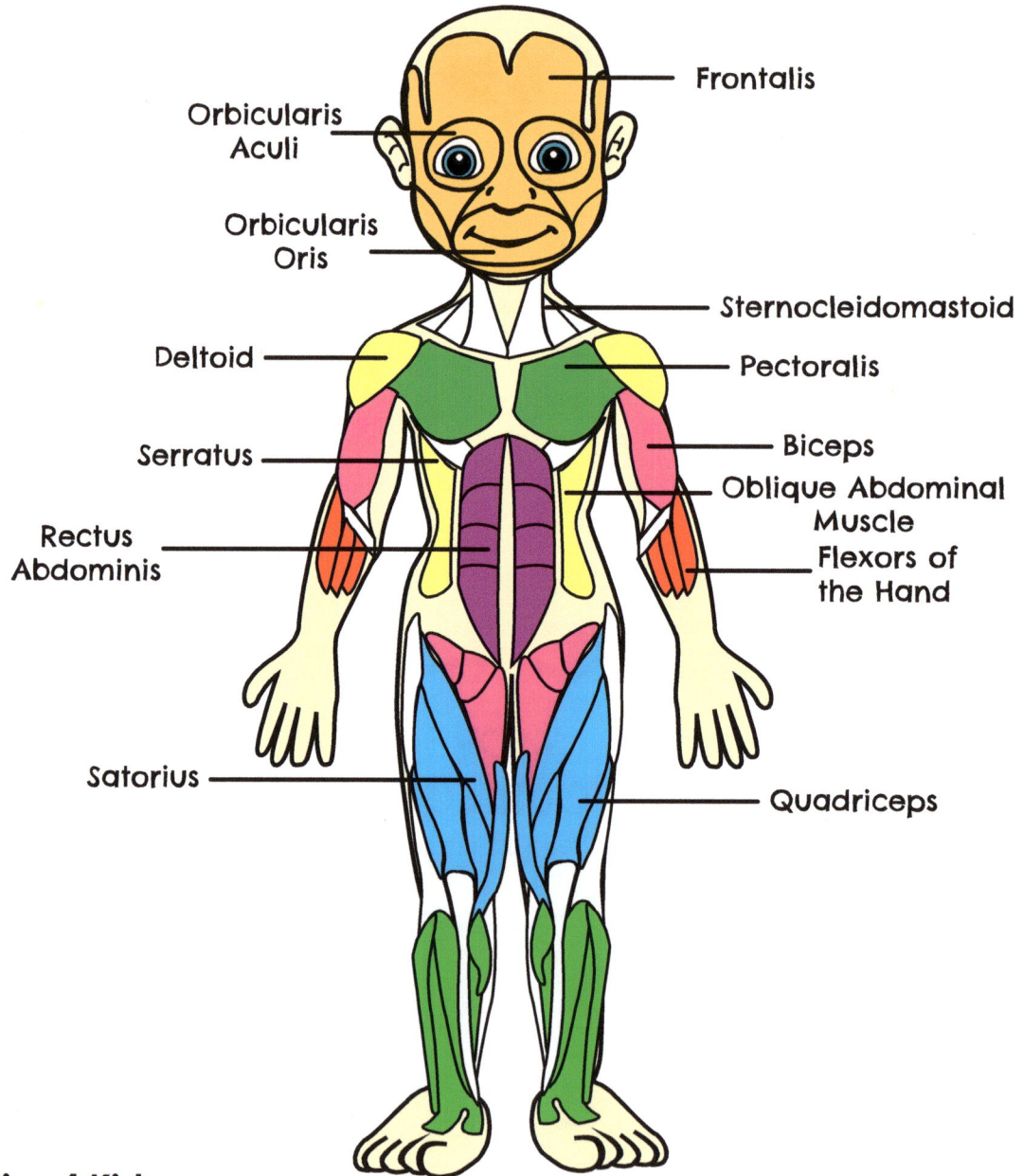

Anatomy

Frontalis

Orbicularis Aculi

Orbicularis Oris

Sternocleidomastoid

Deltoid

Pectoralis

Serratus

Biceps

Oblique Abdominal Muscle

Rectus Abdominis

Flexors of the Hand

Satorius

Quadriceps

Anatomy

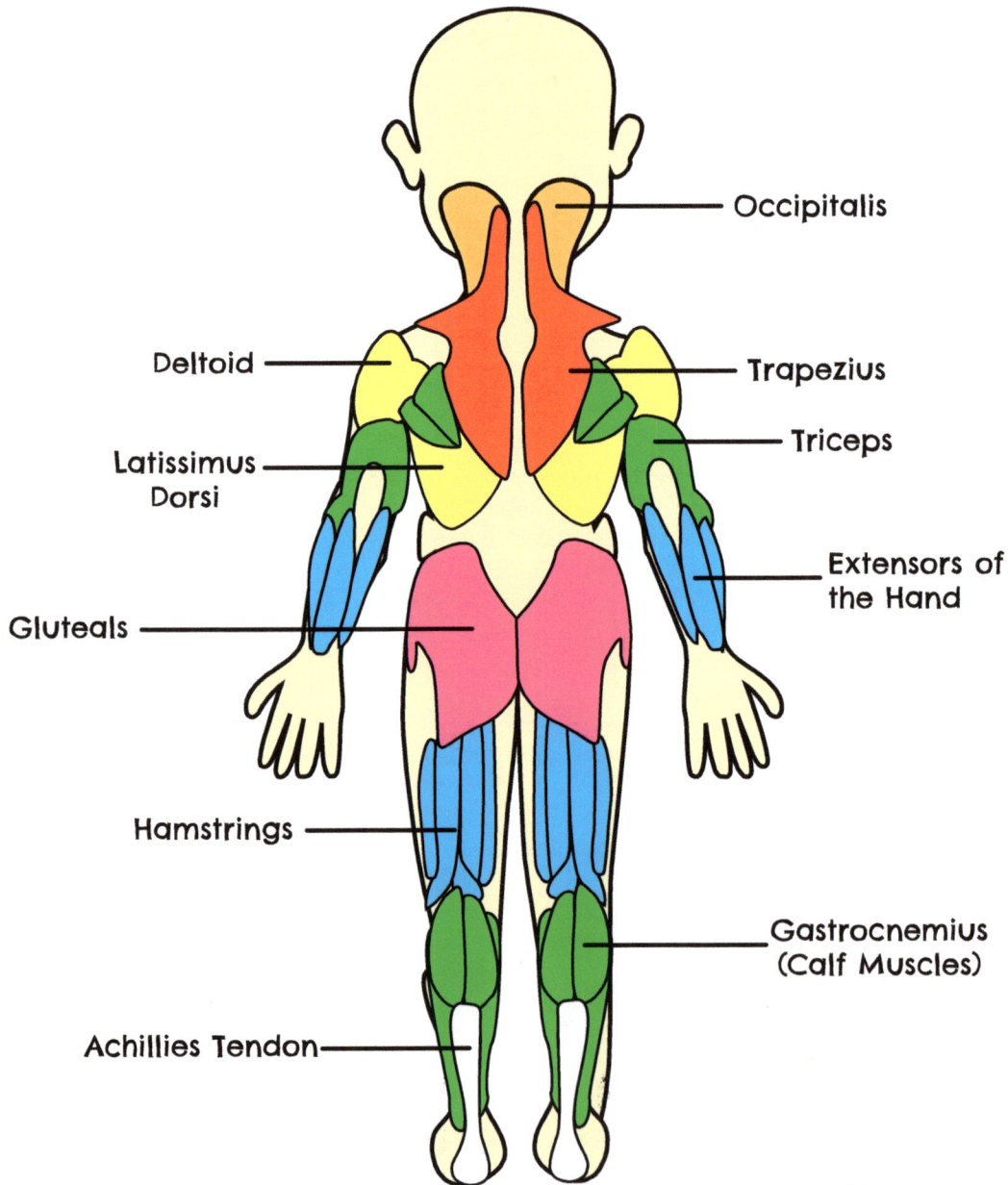

Occipitalis

Deltoid

Trapezius

Triceps

Latissimus Dorsi

Gluteals

Extensors of the Hand

Hamstrings

Gastrocnemius (Calf Muscles)

Achillies Tendon

Catching

Stand up tall

Hold your arms and hands out in front of you

Have your elbows a little bent

Keep your eye on the ball

Reach your arms out in front of you

Catch the ball with both hands

How many can you catch in a row?

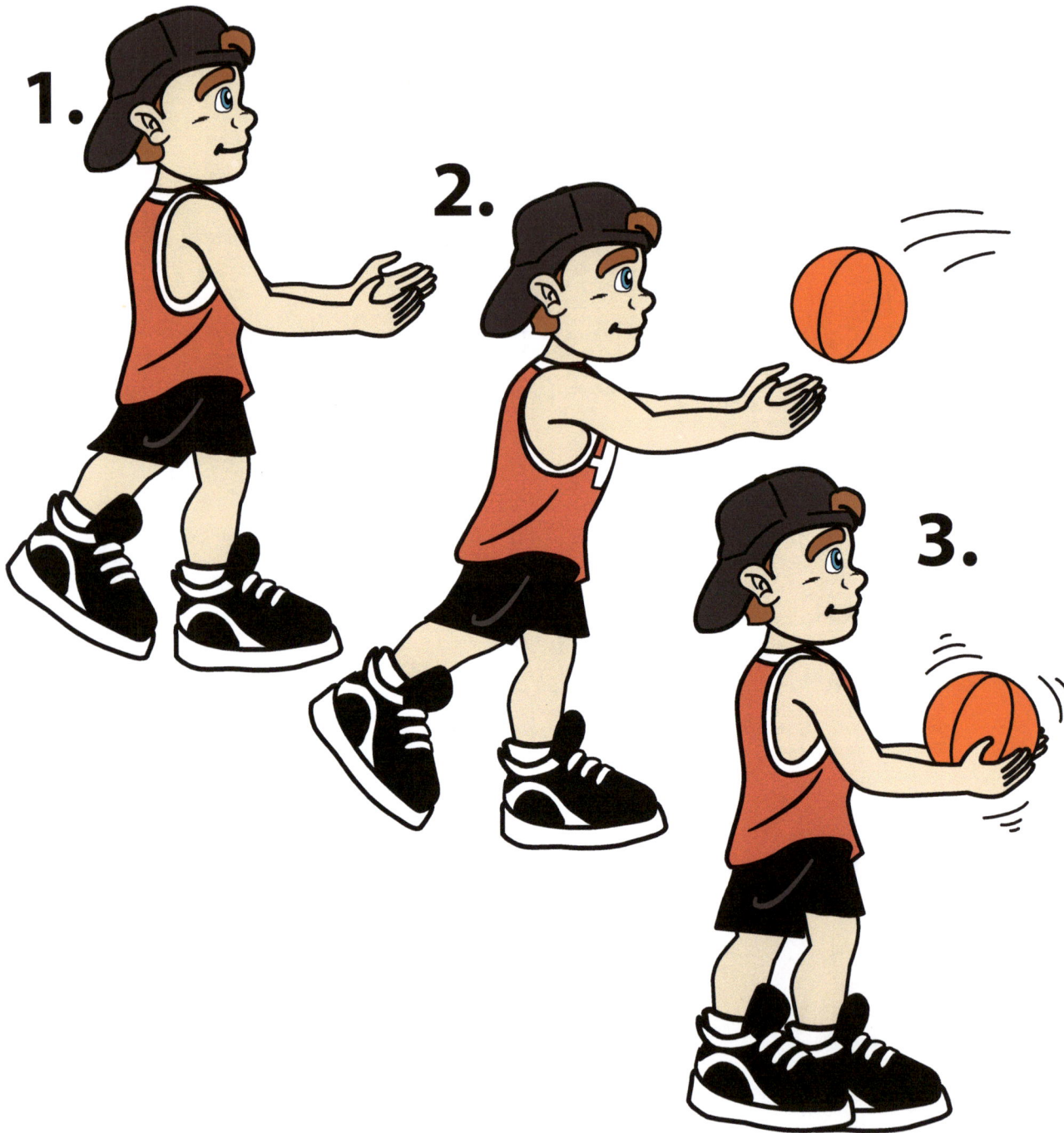

1.

2.

3.

Striking A Stationery Ball

Choose your strongest hand
Place your strong hand above the other
hand when you hold your bat
Turn your body so your leg opposite to
your strong arm is forward
Stand with your feet apart
Move your hips and shoulders around
when swinging the bat
Place all your bodyweight in your back
foot then move it to your front foot when
swinging the bat
Swing the bat and aim to hit the ball
How far can you hit the ball?

1.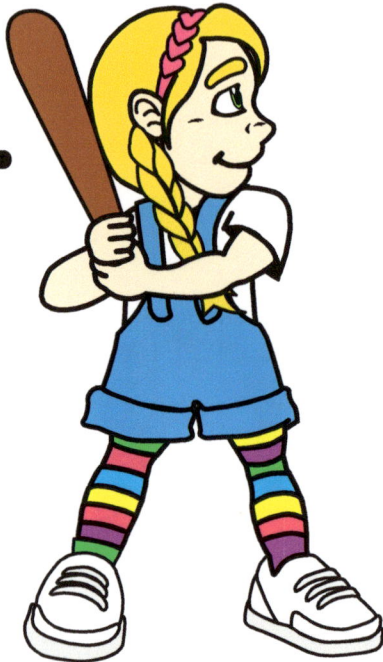

2.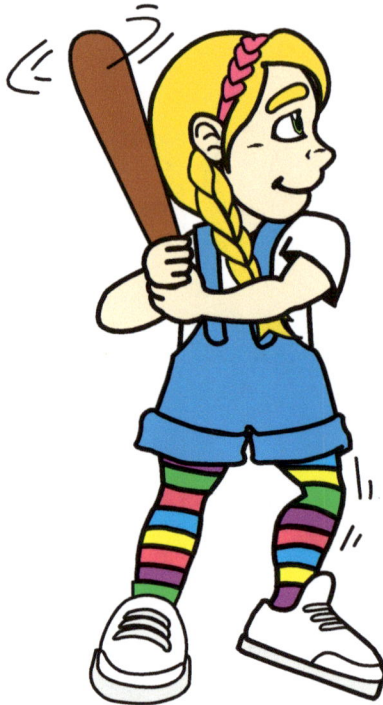

3.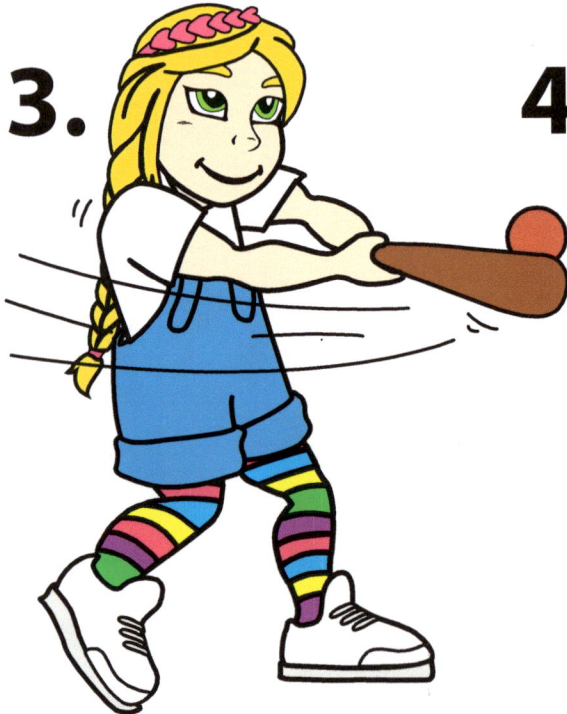

4.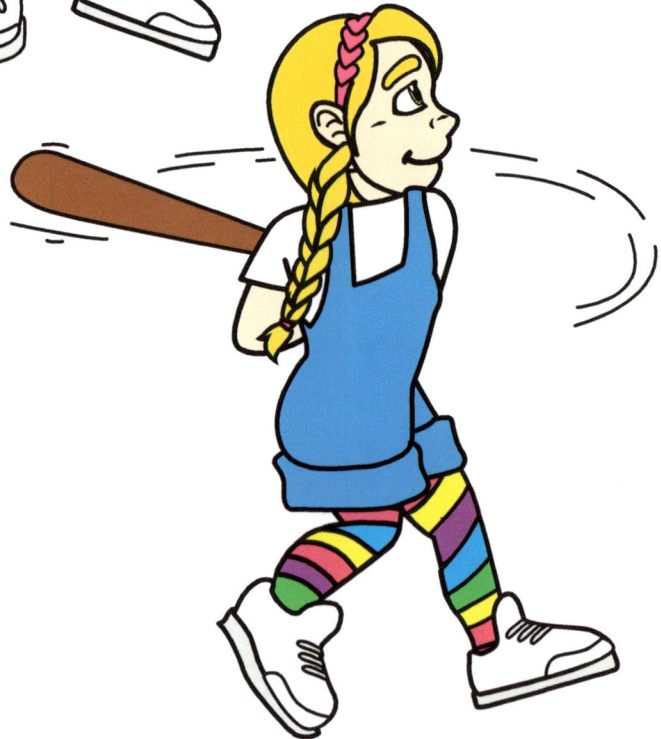

Hopping

Stand up straight and try to balance on one leg

Bend your arms and start to swing them

forward and backwards

When your arms are back bend your

straight leg a little at the knee

Swing your arms forward and take a

hop at the same time

Can you hop 5 times on each leg?

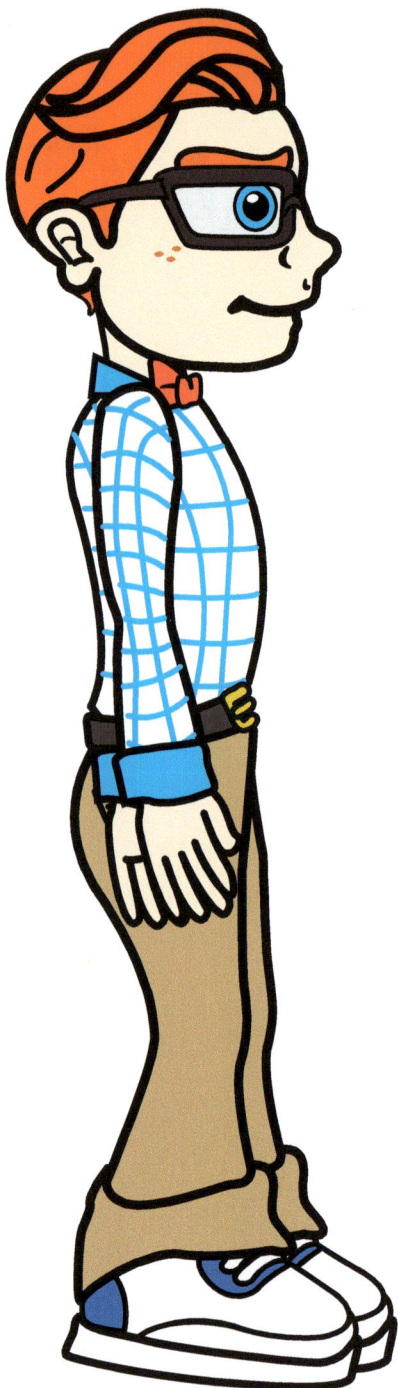

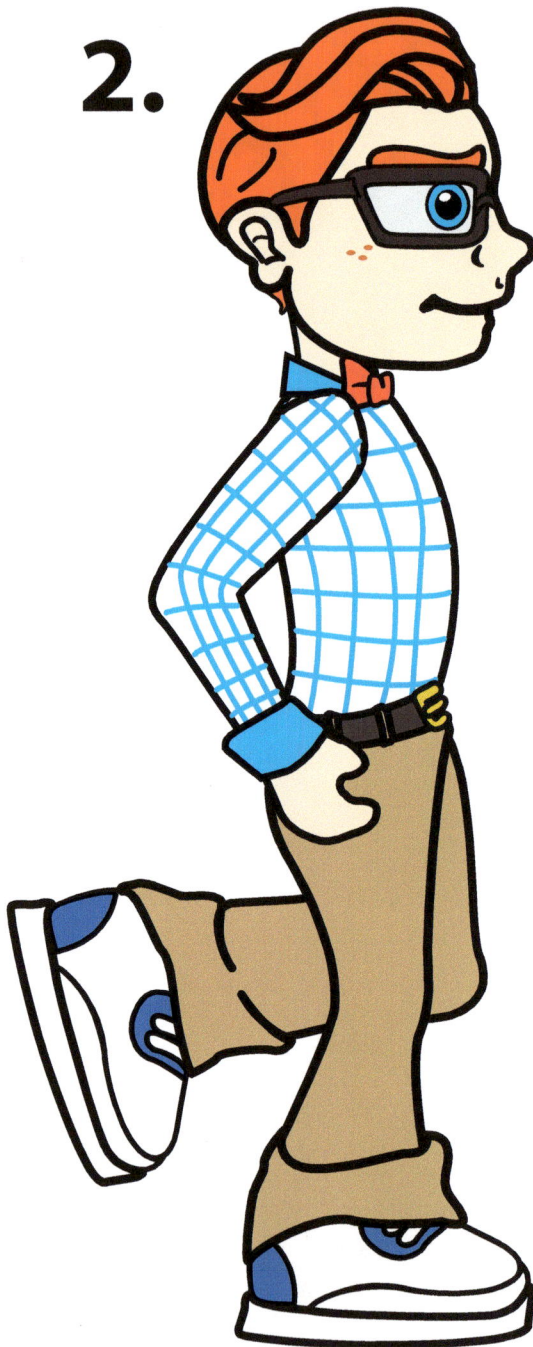

1.

2.

Side Sliding

Stand up straight and turn
your body side ways
With your front leg take
a step side ways
Slide your other leg to meet
your front leg
Can you side slide 5 times
with each leg?

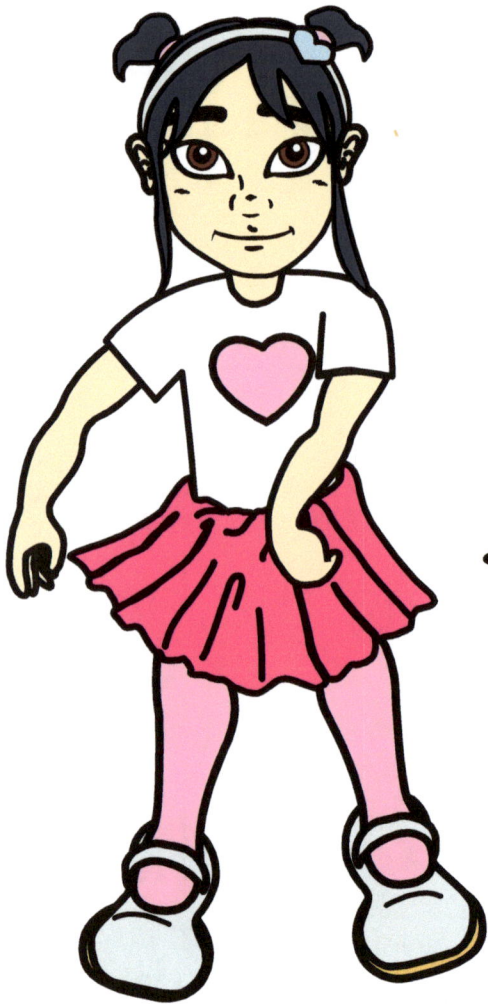
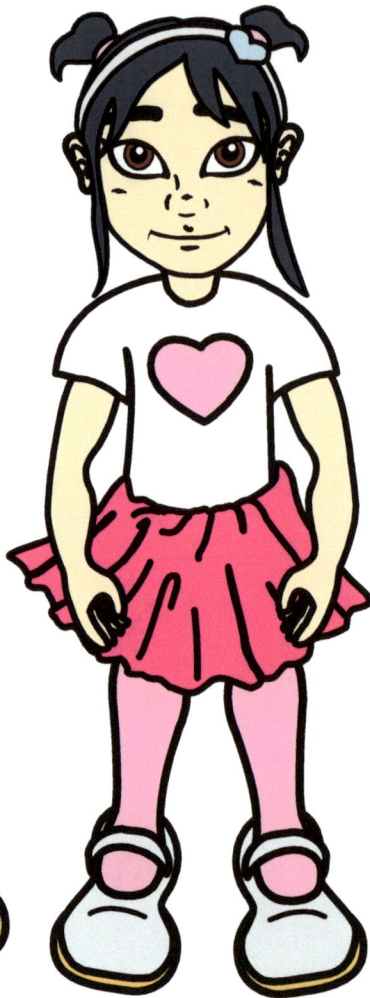
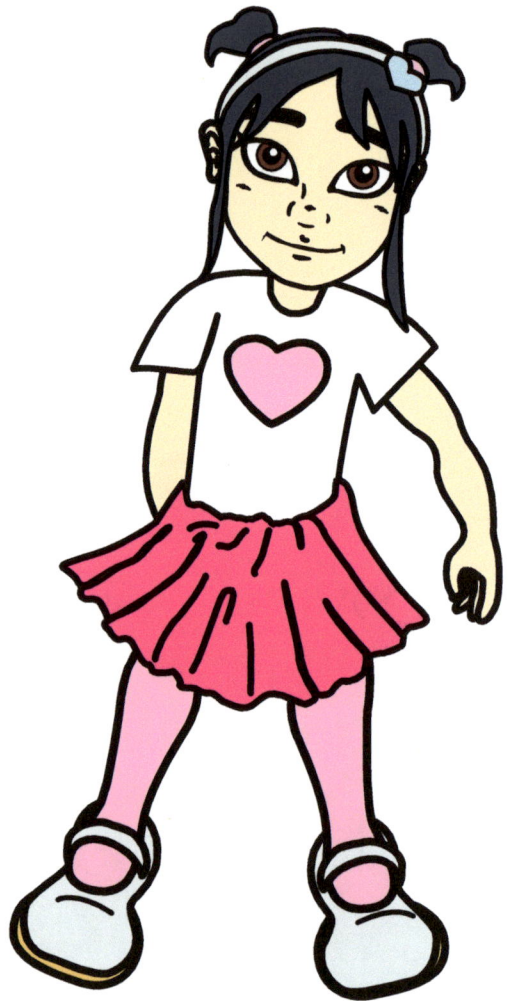

1.

2.

3.

Underarm Rolling

Stand up and hold a ball with one hand

Take a step forward with your opposite leg

Swing your arm back holding the ball

Bend your knees and lower your body

Swing your arm forward and let go of the ball

How far can you get the ball to go?

1.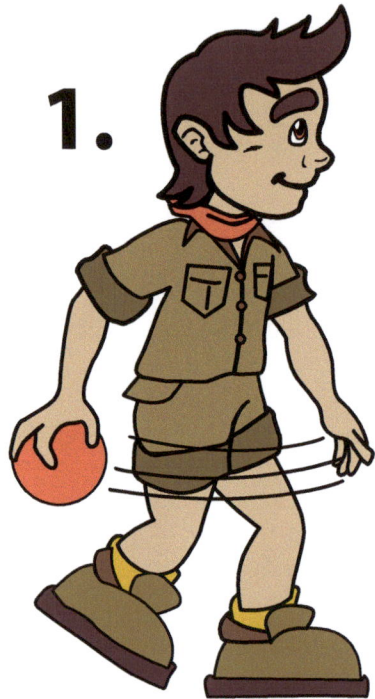

2.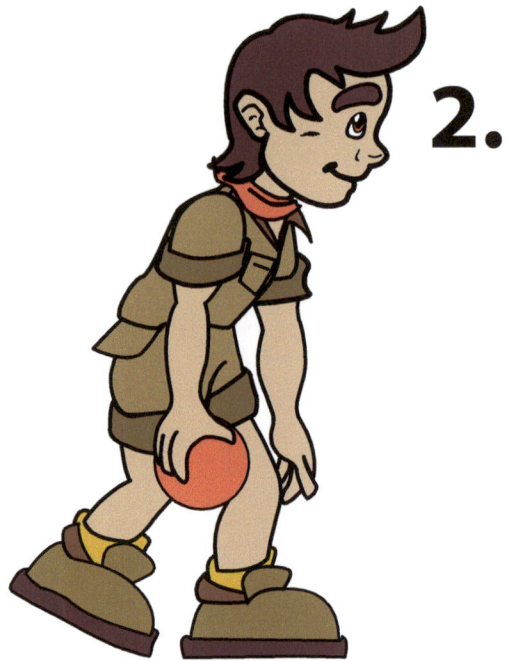

3.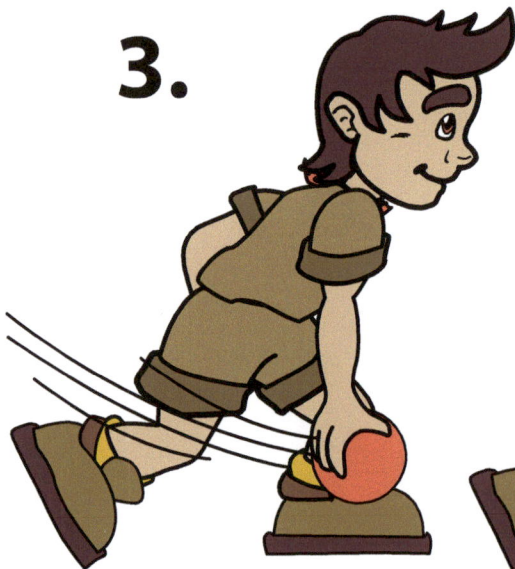

4.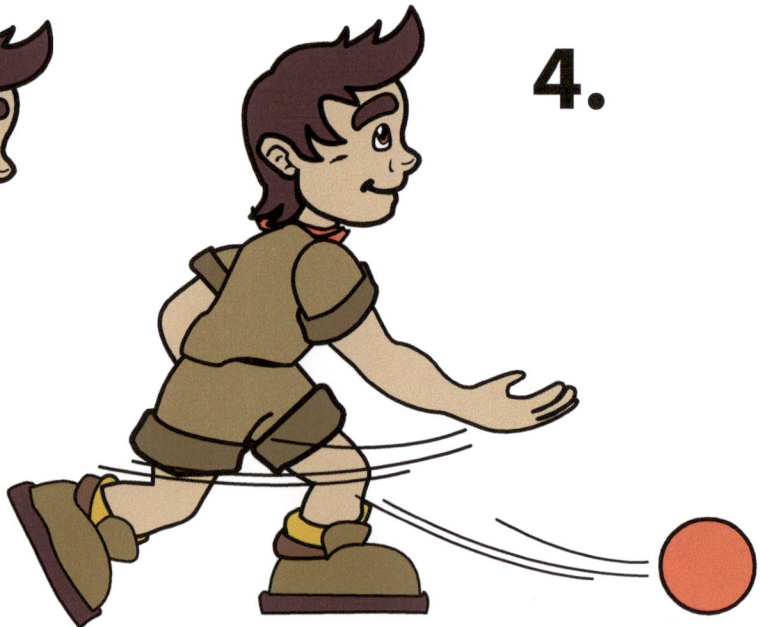

Stationery Dribbling

Stand up and hold the ball with one hand

Using your fingertips push the ball

down onto the ground

Make sure the ball bounces down

in front of your feet

When the ball comes back up push

the ball down again

How many bounces can you do

without stopping?

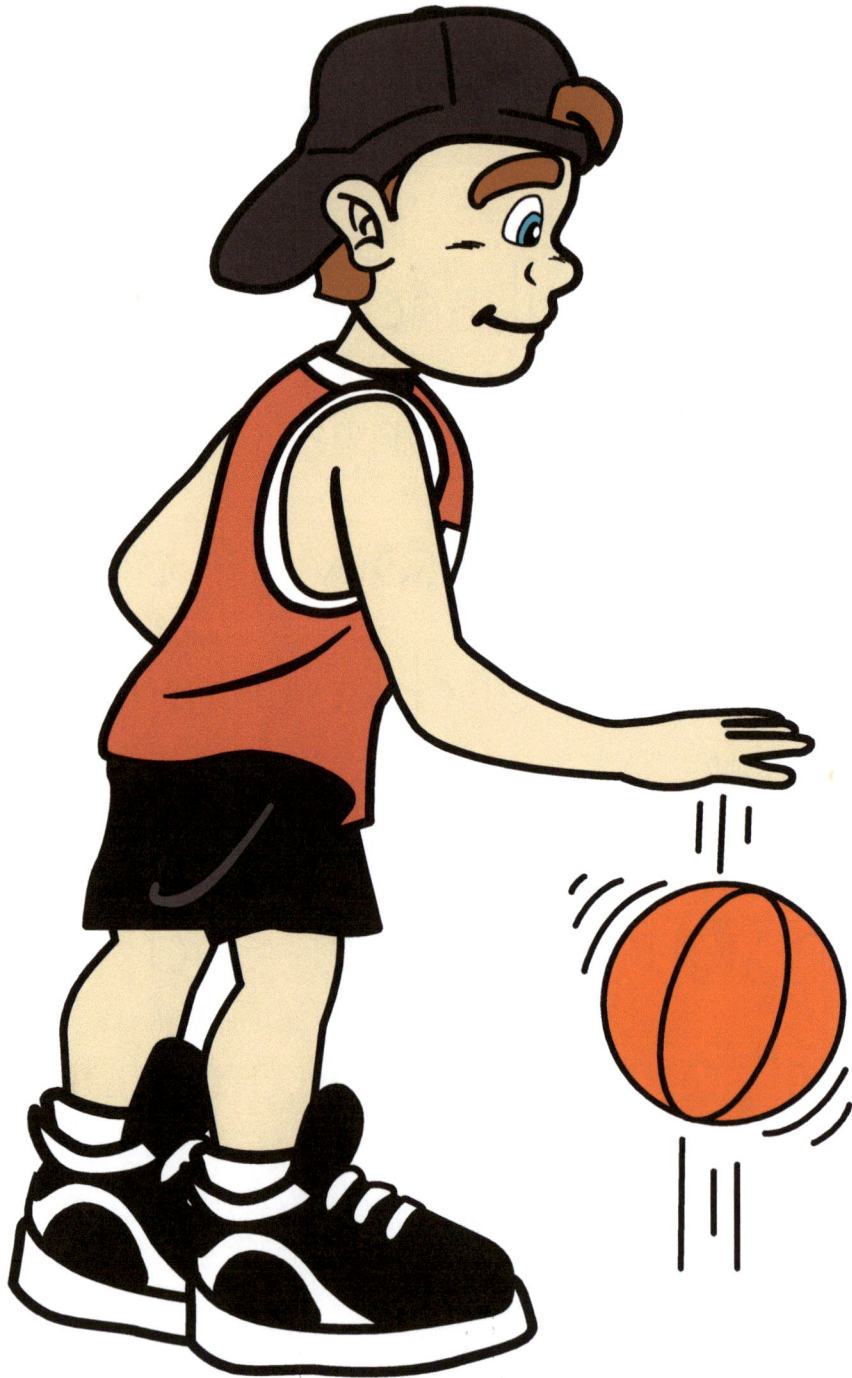

Overarm Throwing

Stand up tall and hold a ball with
your strongest hand
Turn your body so your opposite leg
is forward and your arm is back
Move your body weight to rest on your back leg
When your ready aim and throw your
ball bringing your arm forward
Can you aim and throw at a target
with your ball?

1.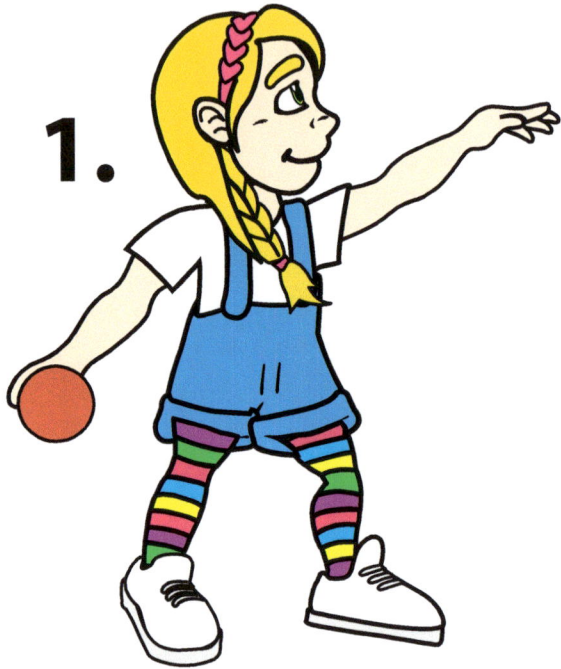

2.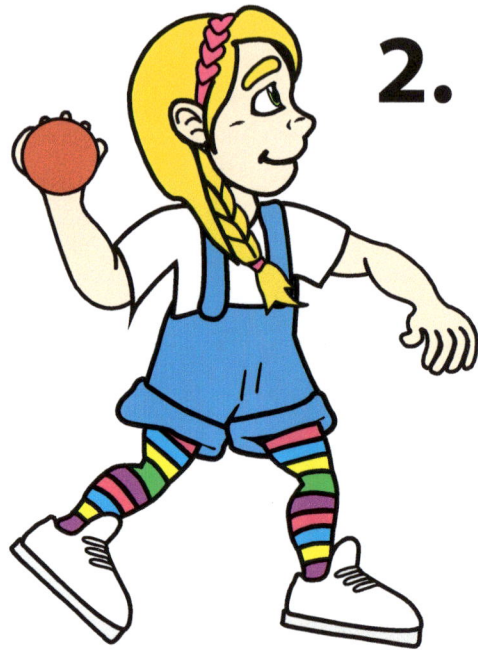

3.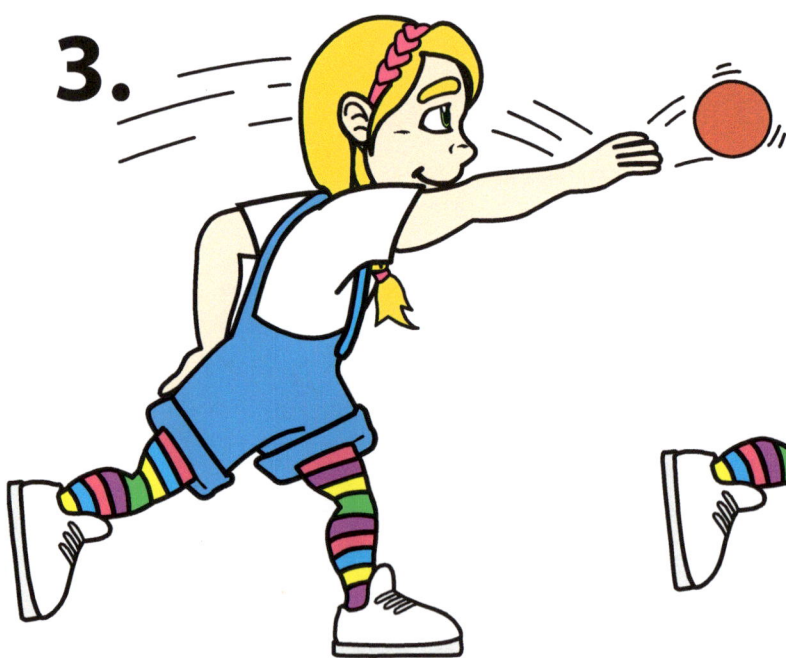

4.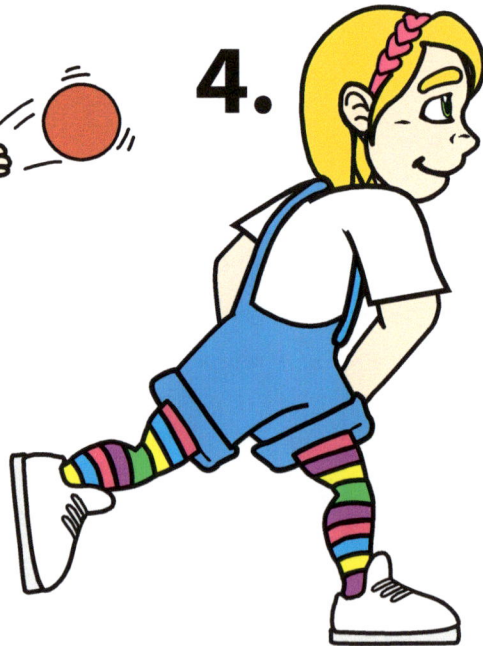

Walking

Let's find a big space

Stand with your body straight

Start slowly swinging your arms by your side

Start to lift your feet

Take small steps forward one leg at a time

Can you walk every day for at least
10 minutes?

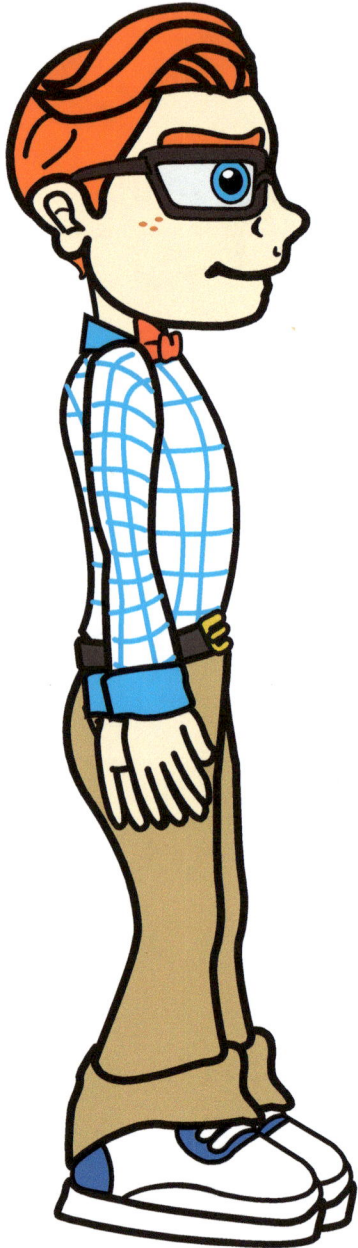

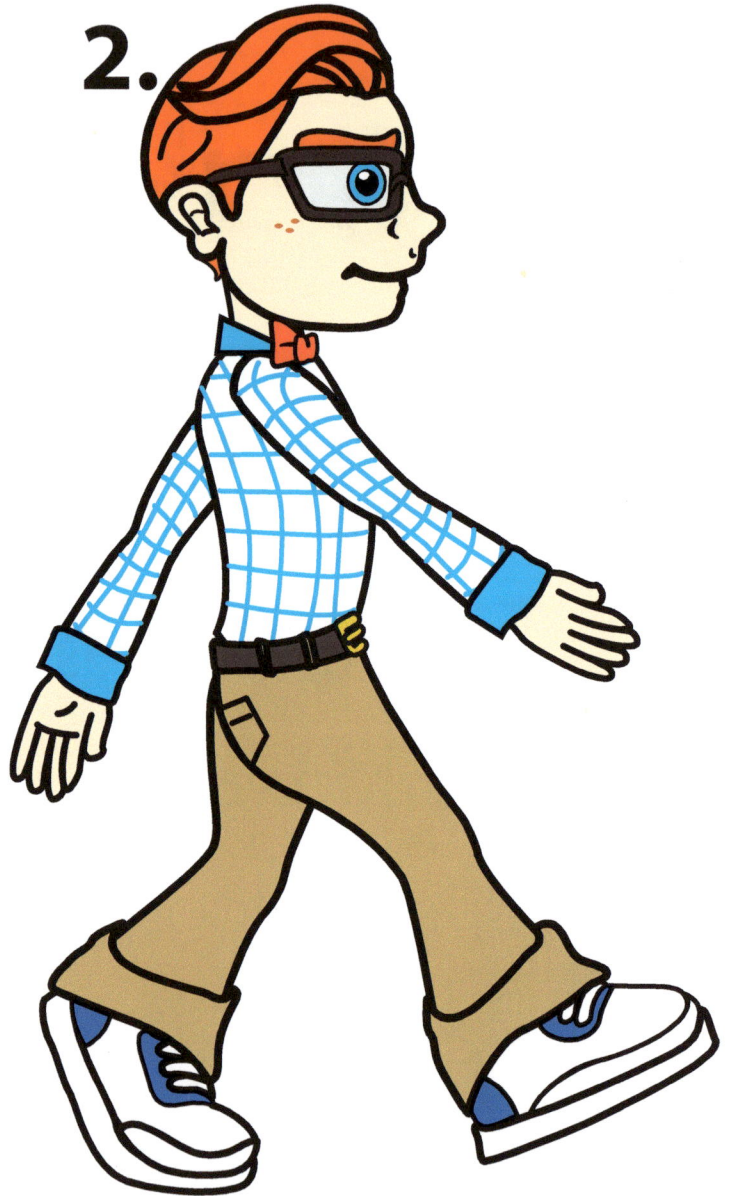

1.

2.

Galloping

Stand up tall

Bend your arms and lift them to

your hips as you take off

Step forward with your first foot

Let your other foot step beside your first foot

Repeat this step slowly at first

Now try gallop faster and faster

1.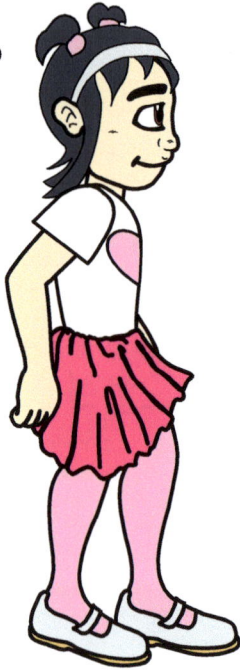

2.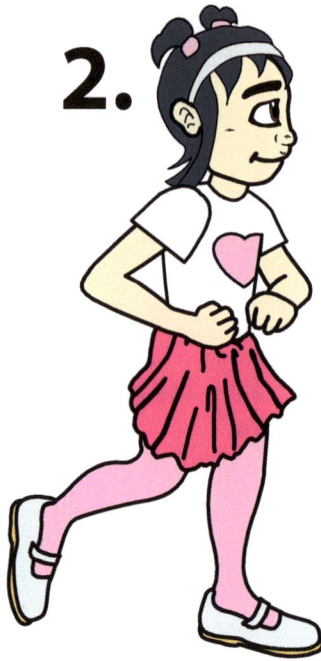

3.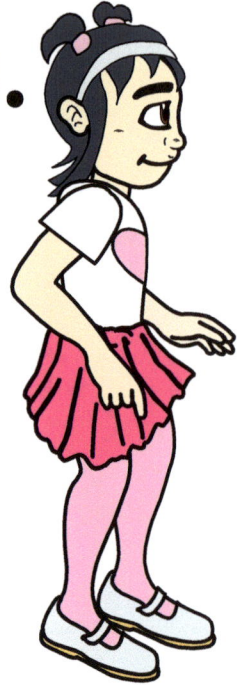

4.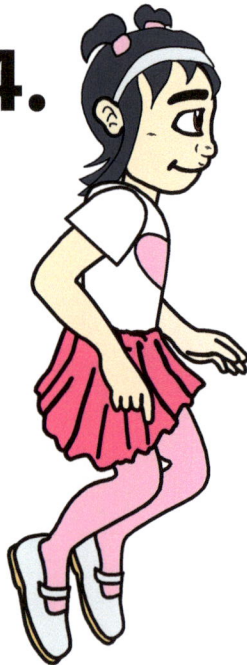

5.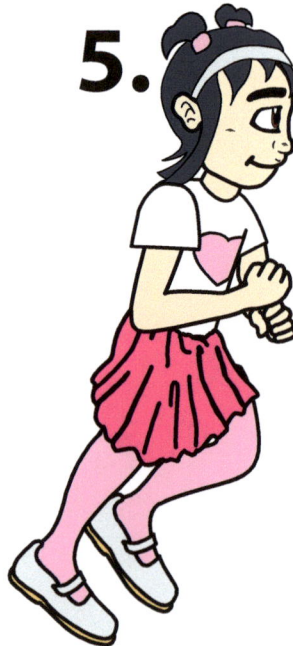

Jumping

Stand up and bend at the knees
Swing your arms backwards
and get ready to jump
Swing your arms forward and upward
Keep them swinging and take off
with both feet and jump
Land with both feet on the floor
Bring your arms down as you land
Can you jump forward 10 times?

1.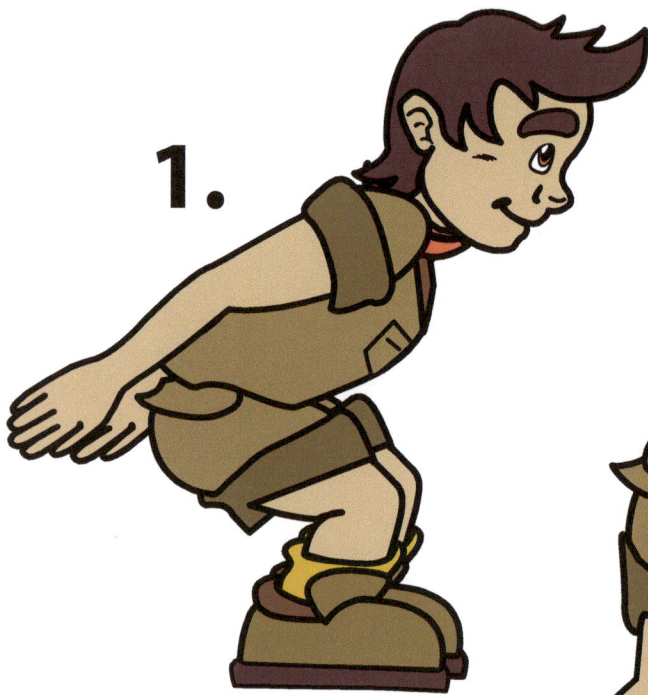

2.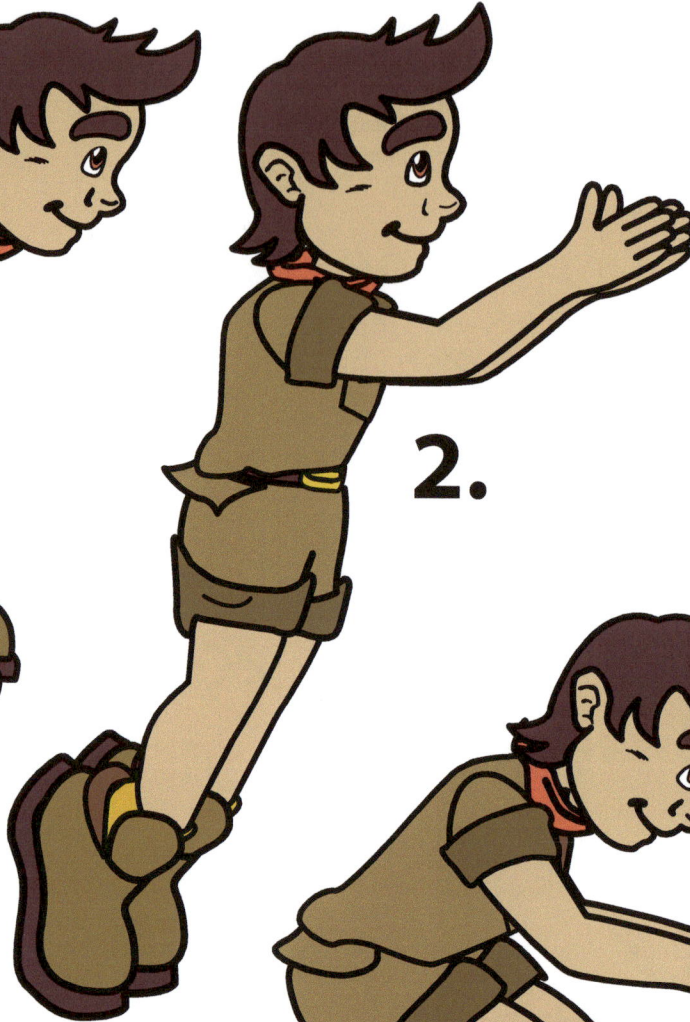

3.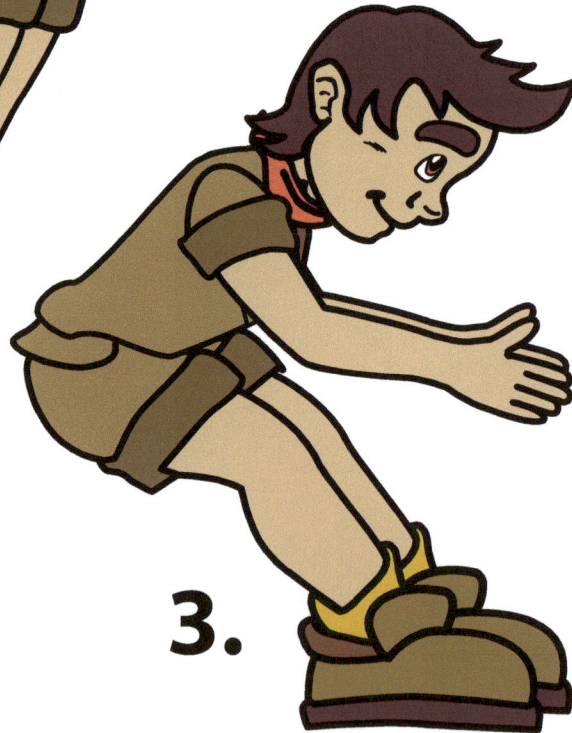

Bending To Squat

Stand up straight near the object you
need to pick up
Bend down slowly at the hips and knees
Keep your back straight at the same time
Slowly lift the object by straightening
your hips and knees
Once your up hold the object close to
your body as high as your belly
Let your feet take you in the direction you
need taking small steps
Try putting the object down again using
the same steps backwards

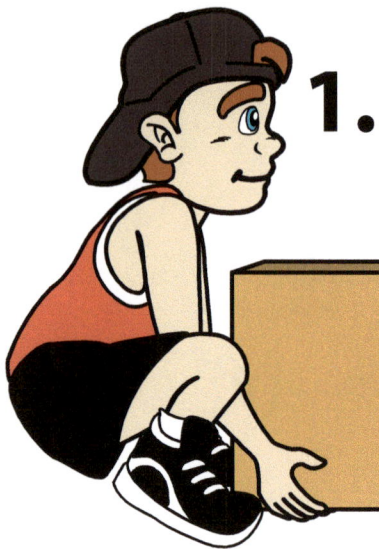

1.

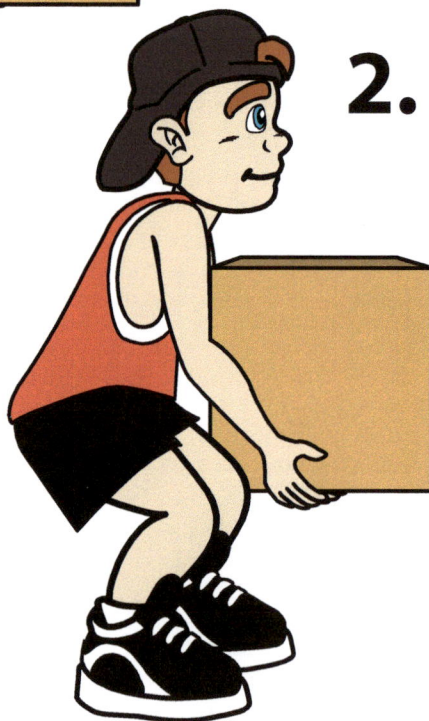

2.

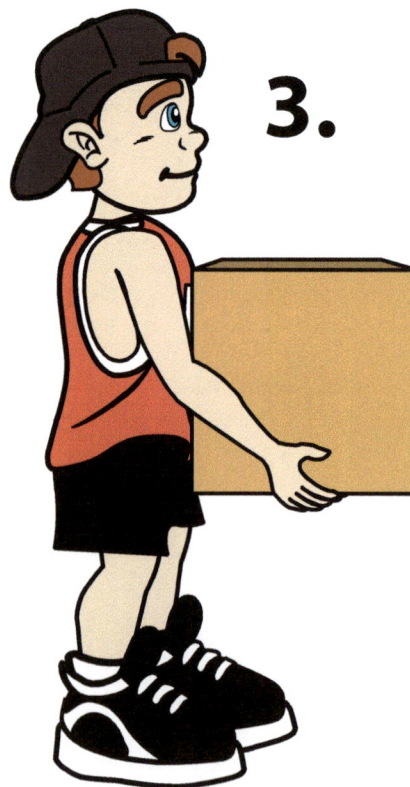

3.

Kicking

Place a ball on the floor in front of you
Take 4 steps back away from the ball
Start to run towards the ball
Just before you get to the ball take a long step forward with one leg
Swing your other leg backwards and get ready to kick
Swing that leg forward and aim and kick the ball with your toes or the top of your foot
How far can you kick the ball?

1.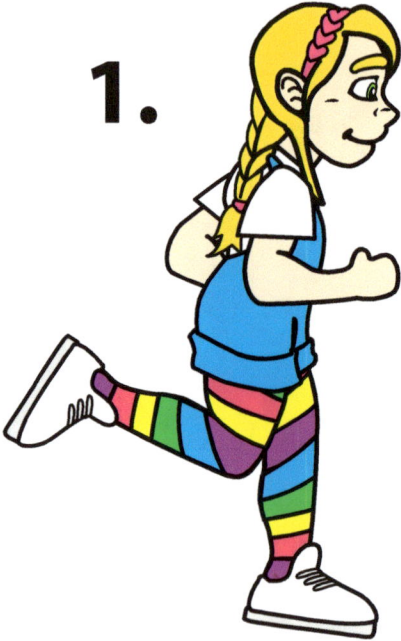

2.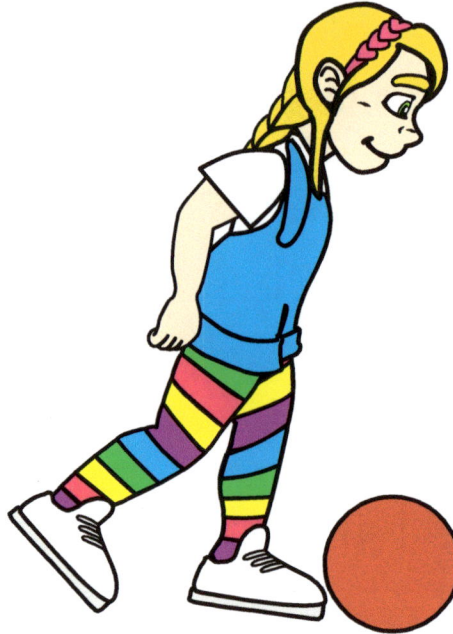

3.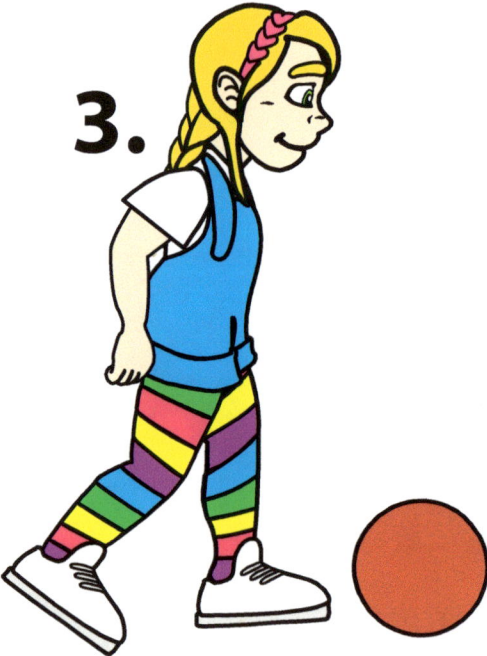

4.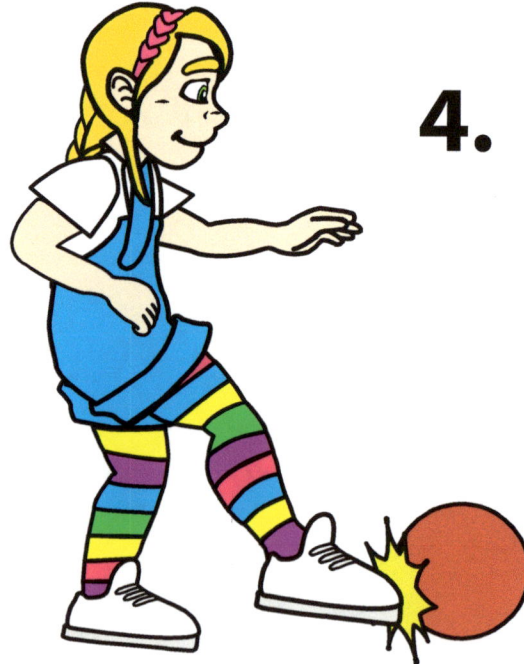

Skipping

Let's grab our rope

Hold an end at each side with our hands

Stand up tall and place your feet together

Place the rope behind your feet

Now swing your rope up around your whole body

When the rope gets back near your feet

take a big jump over the rope

How many jumps can you do

without stopping?

1.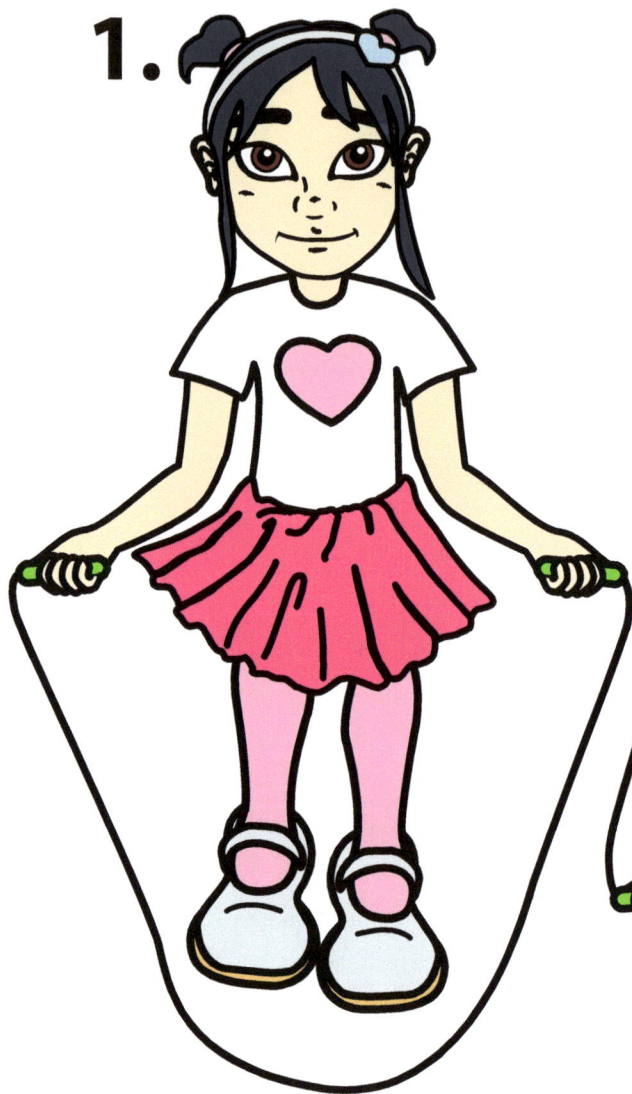

2.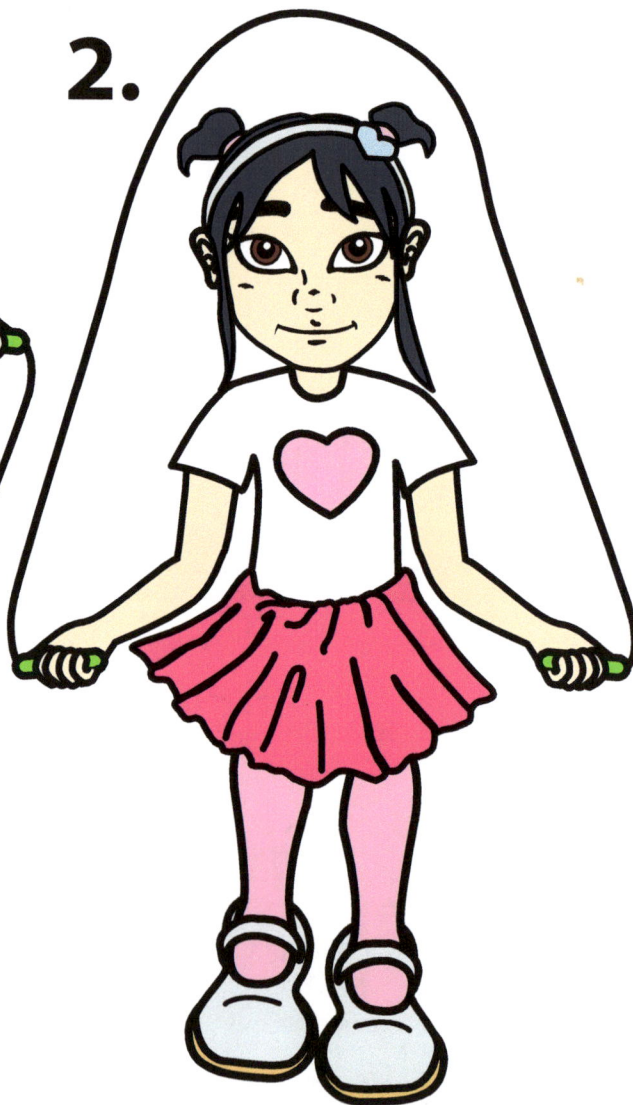

Leaping

Stand up straight

Take a short run off

With one foot take off with a long step

Your body should lift off the ground

Land with your opposite foot

beside your take off foot

Swinging your arms when you leap in

the air will help you leap further

How far can you leap?

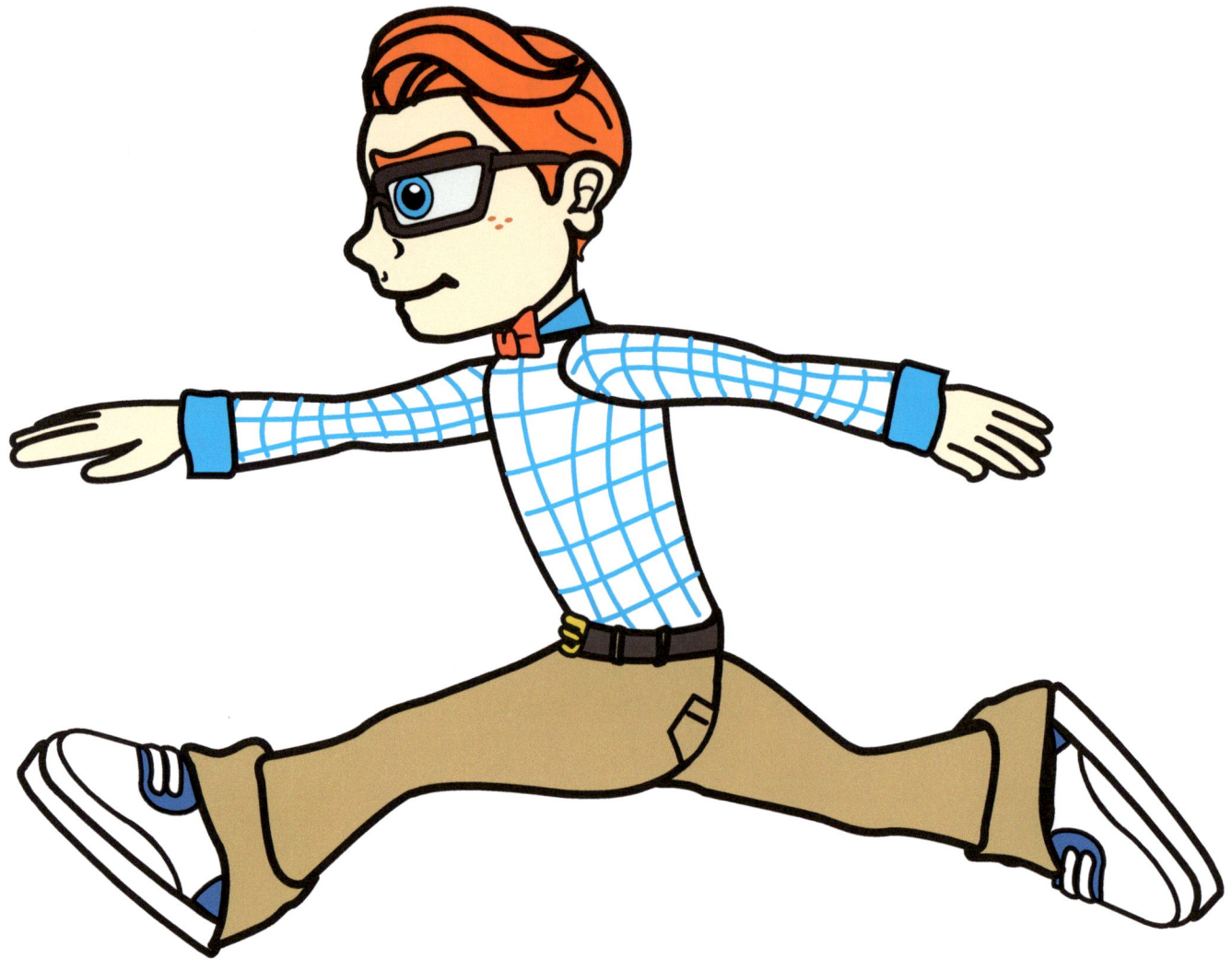

Running

Let's find a big space
Stand with your body straight
Bend your elbows
Start swinging them by your side hip to chin
Start to lift your knees and feet one at a time
Now start to take a step forward
with each leg
Lets see how fast you can run

1.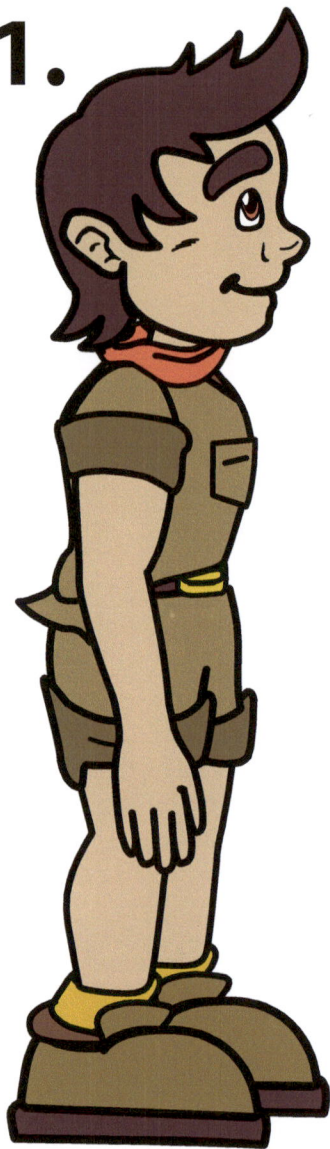

2.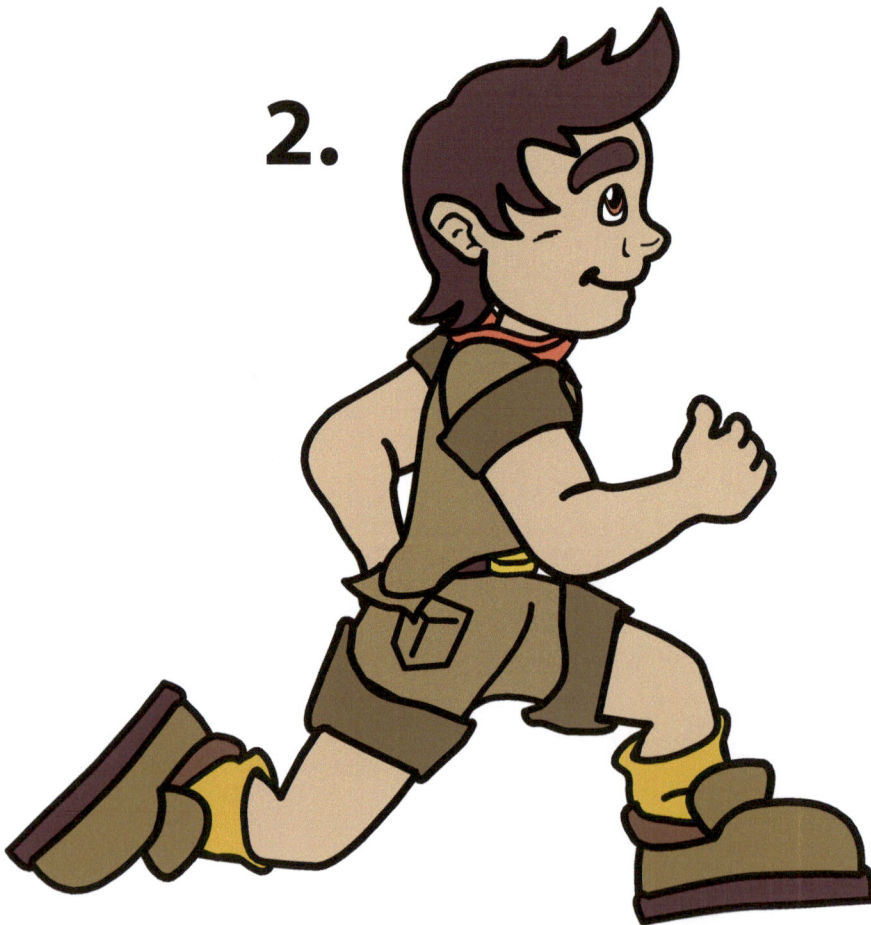

Keep an eye out for the rest of the series

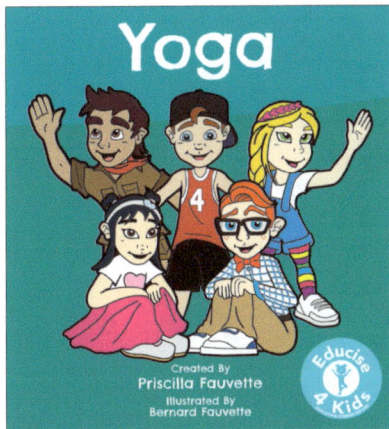

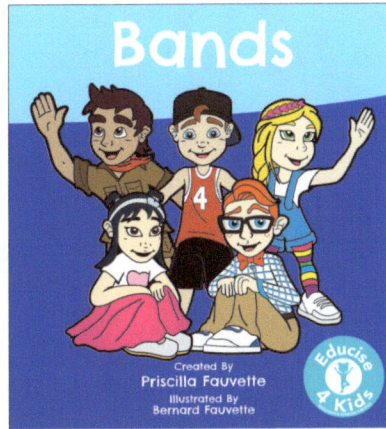

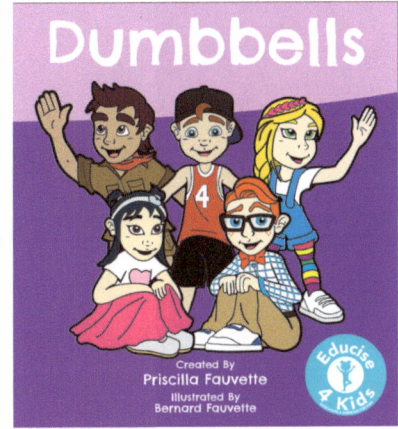

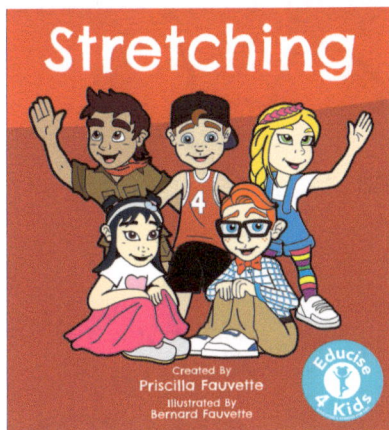

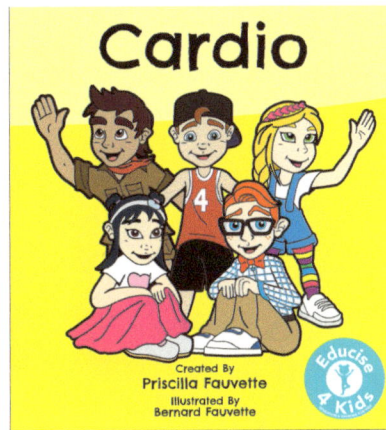

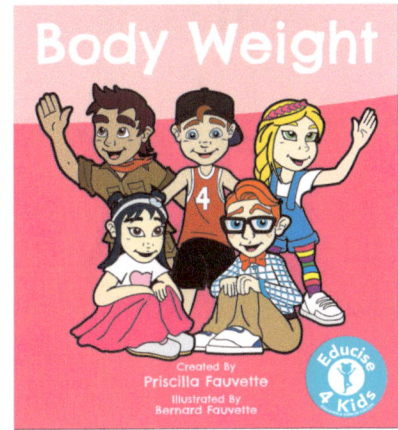

Yoga

Created By
Priscilla Fauvette
Illustrated By
Bernard Fauvette

Educise 4 Kids

Bands

Created By
Priscilla Fauvette
Illustrated By
Bernard Fauvette

Educise 4 Kids

Dumbbells

Created By
Priscilla Fauvette
Illustrated By
Bernard Fauvette

Educise 4 Kids

Stretching

Created By
Priscilla Fauvette
Illustrated By
Bernard Fauvette

Educise 4 Kids

Cardio

Created By
Priscilla Fauvette
Illustrated By
Bernard Fauvette

Educise 4 Kids

Body Weight

Created By
Priscilla Fauvette
Illustrated By
Bernard Fauvette

Educise 4 Kids

www.ingramcontent.com/pod-product-compliance
Lightning Source LLC
Chambersburg PA
CBHW061137030426
42334CB00003B/79